DELICIOUS CABBAGE RECIPE COOKBOOK

20 easy and mouth-watering Trusted cabbage recipes

Jennifer J. Rodriguez

Table of content

INTRODUCTION

Welcome to the world of delectable flavors and wholesome goodness! In our "Delicious Cabbage Recipe Cookbook," we invite you to embark on a culinary adventure where the humble cabbage takes center stage. Bursting with versatile possibilities and nutritional benefits, this cookbook is your ultimate guide to discovering the incredible potential of this underrated vegetable.

Within these pages, you'll find a treasure trove of mouthwatering recipes that showcase the cabbage's remarkable ability to transform any dish into a culinary masterpiece. From refreshing salads and comforting soups to hearty main courses and delightful side dishes, our cookbook presents a diverse array of cabbage-centric recipes to tantalize your taste buds and elevate your meals to new heights.

Whether you're a seasoned chef looking to explore innovative recipes or a cooking enthusiast eager to add a healthy twist to your meals, this cookbook is designed to inspire and guide you every step of the way. With clear instructions, helpful tips, and stunning visuals, you'll embark on a culinary journey that embraces the flavors, textures, and endless possibilities that cabbage has to offer.

Beyond its incredible taste and culinary versatility, cabbage boasts an array of health benefits. Packed with vitamins, minerals, and antioxidants, this cruciferous vegetable has long been celebrated for its ability to support a well-rounded and nutritious diet. With our recipes, you'll discover how cabbage can effortlessly enhance the nutritional value of your meals while ensuring they remain irresistibly delicious.

So, whether you're craving a comforting bowl of cabbage soup on a chilly evening, seeking a zesty coleslaw to brighten up your summer barbecues, or eager to explore exciting new cabbage-based creations, our "Delicious Cabbage Recipe Cookbook" is here to guide you on a flavorful journey. Prepare to unlock the culinary potential of cabbage and discover a world of taste sensations that will leave you craving more. Get ready to turn the ordinary into the extraordinary, one cabbage recipe at a time!

DELICIOUS CABBAGE RECIPE

HEARTY MAIN COURSES

1. Stuffed Cabbage Rolls

Ingredients:
- 1 large cabbage head
- 1 pound ground beef
- 1 cup cooked rice
- 1 onion, finely chopped
- 2 cloves garlic, minced
- 1 can tomato sauce
- Salt and pepper to taste
- 1 tablespoon olive oil

Instructions:
- Preheat the oven to 350°F (175°C).
- Carefully remove the cabbage leaves and blanch them in boiling water for 2-3 minutes. Drain and set aside.
- In a bowl, mix the ground beef, cooked rice, onion, garlic, salt, and pepper.
- Place a spoonful of the beef mixture onto each cabbage leaf and roll them tightly.
- Place the stuffed cabbage rolls in a baking dish, pour tomato sauce over them, and drizzle with olive oil.za- Bake the dish for 45 minutes

with the foil covering it. After 15 minutes, take the foil off and bake the dish until golden brown.

2. Cabbage And Sausage Stir-Fry

Ingredients:
- 1 small cabbage, thinly sliced
- 1 pound sausage, sliced
- 1 red bell pepper, sliced
- 1 onion, sliced
- 2 cloves garlic, minced
- 2 tablespoons soy sauce
- 1 tablespoon oyster sauce
- 1 tablespoon sesame oil
- Salt and pepper to taste

Instructions:
- Over medium heat, warm the sesame oil in a sizable skillet or wok.
- Sausage slices should be added and cooked until browned.
- Add the onion, garlic, and red bell pepper to the skillet and stir-fry for 2-3 minutes.
- Add the cabbage and continue to stir-fry for another 5-7 minutes until the cabbage is tender-crisp.
- Whisk soy sauce and oyster sauce together in a small bowl. Pour the sauce over the cabbage mixture and toss to coat evenly.

- Season with salt and pepper to taste. Serve hot.

3. Cabbage And Potato Casserole

Ingredients:
- 1 medium cabbage, shredded
- Peeled and thinly sliced four medium potatoes
- 1 onion, thinly sliced
- 1 cup shredded cheddar cheese
- 1 cup milk
- 2 tablespoons butter
- Salt and pepper to taste

Instructions:
- Preheat the oven to 375°F (190°C). Grease a baking dish with butter.
- Layer half of the cabbage, potatoes, and onion in the baking dish. Sprinkle it with salt and pepper.
- Repeat the layers with the remaining cabbage, potatoes, and onion. Sprinkle it with salt and pepper again.
- Pour the milk over the layers and top with shredded cheddar cheese.
- Dot the top with butter and cover the dish with foil.
- Bake for 45 minutes. Remove the foil and bake for an additional 15-20 minutes until the

top is golden brown and the potatoes are tender. Serve warm.

4. Cabbage And Beef Stir-Fry

Ingredients:
- 1 small cabbage, shredded
- 1 pound beef sirloin, thinly sliced
- 1 onion, sliced
- 2 carrots, julienned
- 2 cloves garlic, minced
- 2 tablespoons soy sauce
- 1 tablespoon oyster sauce
- 1 tablespoon vegetable oil
- Salt and pepper to taste

Instructions:
- In a sizable skillet or wok, heat vegetable oil over high heat.
- Add the sliced beef and cook until browned. From the skillet, take out the beef, and set it aside.
- In the same skillet, add the onion, carrots, and minced garlic. Vegetables should be stir-fried for 2–3 minutes until crisp-tender.
- Add the shredded cabbage to the skillet and continue to stir-fry for another 3-4 minutes until the cabbage wilts.

- Return the beef to the skillet and stir in the soy sauce and oyster sauce. Toss to coat everything evenly.
- Season with salt and pepper to taste. Cook for another 2-3 minutes to thoroughly cook everything.
- Remove from heat and serve hot.

5. Cabbage Roll Casserole:

Ingredients:
- 1 small cabbage, shredded
- 1 pound ground beef
- 1 onion, diced
- 2 cloves garlic, minced
- 1 cup cooked rice
- 1 can diced tomatoes
- 1 can tomato sauce
- 1 tablespoon Worcestershire sauce
- 1 teaspoon dried oregano
- 1 teaspoon dried basil
- Salt and pepper to taste
- 1 cup shredded mozzarella cheese

Instructions:
- Preheat the oven to 375°F (190°C). Grease a casserole dish.
- In a large skillet, cook the ground beef, onion, and minced garlic over medium heat until the beef is browned. Drain any excess fat.

- Stir in the cooked rice, diced tomatoes, tomato sauce, Worcestershire sauce, dried oregano, dried basil, salt, and pepper. Cook for 5 minutes to combine the flavors.
- Layer half of the shredded cabbage in the casserole dish. Place half of the beef mixture on top.
- Repeat the layers with the remaining cabbage and beef mixture.
- Top with the shredded mozzarella cheese.
- Bake for 45 minutes, covered with foil.
- Remove the cover and bake for another 10-15 minutes, or until the cheese is bubbling and brown.
- Let it cool slightly before serving.

6. Cabbage And Chicken Stir-Fry

Ingredients:
- 1 small cabbage, thinly sliced
- 2 thinly sliced boneless, skinless chicken breasts
- 1 bell pepper, sliced
- 1 carrot, julienned
- 2 cloves garlic, minced
- 2 tablespoons soy sauce
- 1 tablespoon hoisin sauce
- 1 tablespoon sesame oil
- 1 tablespoon vegetable oil
- Salt and pepper to taste

Instructions:

- In a large skillet or wok, heat the vegetable oil over high heat.
- Cook until the sliced chicken is browned and cooked through. Set the chicken aside after removing it from the skillet.
- In the same skillet, add the sliced bell pepper, julienned carrot, and minced garlic. Stir-fry the vegetables for 2-3 minutes, or until they are tender-crisp.
- Add the thinly sliced cabbage to the skillet and continue to stir-fry for another 3-4 minutes until the cabbage wilts.
- Return the chicken to the skillet and stir in the soy sauce, hoisin sauce, and sesame oil. Toss to coat everything evenly.
- Season with salt and pepper to taste. Cook for another 2-3 minutes to thoroughly cook everything.
- Remove from heat and serve hot.

SOUPS:

7. Cabbage And White Bean Soup

Ingredients:
- 1 small cabbage, shredded
- 2 cups cooked white beans
- 1 onion, diced

- 2 carrots, diced
- 2 stalks celery, diced
- 4 cups vegetable broth
- 2 cloves garlic, minced
- 2 tablespoons olive oil
- 1 teaspoon dried thyme
- Salt and pepper to taste

Instructions:
- In a large pot over medium heat, heat the olive oil.
- Add the onion, carrots, celery, and garlic. Cook for 5 minutes, or until the vegetables are soft.
- Stir in the shredded cabbage and cook for another 5 minutes.
- Add the vegetable broth, cooked white beans, and dried thyme. Season with salt and pepper.
- Bring the soup to a boil, then reduce the heat to low and simmer for 20-25 minutes until the cabbage is cooked through and tender.
- Adjust the seasoning if needed. Serve hot.

8. Cabbage And Sausage Soup

Ingredients:
- 1 small cabbage, chopped
- 1 pound smoked sausage, sliced
- 1 onion, diced
- 2 carrots, diced

- 2 stalks celery, diced
- 4 cups chicken broth
- 2 cloves garlic, minced
- 2 tablespoons olive oil
- 1 teaspoon paprika
- Salt and pepper to taste

Instructions:
- In a large pot over medium heat, heat the olive oil.
- Add the onion, carrots, celery, and garlic. Cook for 5 minutes, or until the vegetables are soft.
- Stir in the smoked sausage and cook for another 5 minutes until lightly browned.
- Add the chopped cabbage and paprika. Season with salt and pepper.
- Bring the soup to a boil by adding the chicken broth.
- Reduce the heat to low and simmer for 25-30 minutes until the cabbage is tender.
- Adjust the seasoning if needed. Serve hot.

9. Creamy Cabbage and Potato Soup

Ingredients:
- 1 small cabbage, shredded
- 3 medium potatoes, peeled and diced
- 1 onion, diced
- 4 cups vegetable broth

- 1 cup heavy cream
- 2 tablespoons butter
- 2 cloves garlic, minced
- Salt and pepper to taste

Instructions:
- In a large pot over medium heat, melt the butter.
- Add the onion and garlic. Sauté for 2-3 minutes until the onion is translucent.

- stir in the shredded cabbage and cubed potatoes. Cook for another 5 minutes.
- Pour in the vegetable broth and bring the mixture to a boil.
- Reduce the heat to low, cover the pot, and simmer for 20-25 minutes until the potatoes are tender.

- Using an immersion blender, smooth and creamy the soup.
- Season with salt and pepper and stir in the heavy cream.
- Simmer for an additional 5 minutes until heated through. Serve hot.

10. Cabbage and Lentil Soup

Ingredients:
1 small cabbage, chopped

1 cup green or brown lentils, rinsed
1 onion, diced
2 carrots, diced
2 stalks celery, diced
4 cups vegetable broth
2 cloves garlic, minced
2 tablespoons olive oil
1 teaspoon cumin
1/2 teaspoon paprika
Salt and pepper to taste

Instructions:

- In a big pot, heat olive oil over medium heat.
Mix in the onion, carrots, celery, and garlic. Sauté the vegetables for 5 minutes, or until they are soft.
- Stir in the chopped cabbage and cook for another 5 minutes until it begins to wilt.
- Add the rinsed lentils, cumin, paprika, salt, and pepper to the pot. Stir to combine everything evenly.
- Bring the soup to a boil after adding the veggie broth.
- Reduce the heat to low and simmer for 30-35 minutes until the lentils and cabbage are cooked through.
- Adjust the seasoning if needed. Serve hot.

11. Cabbage and Tomato Soup

Ingredients:
1 small cabbage, shredded
1 onion, diced
2 cloves garlic, minced
1 can diced tomatoes
4 cups vegetable broth
2 tablespoons tomato paste
1 tablespoon olive oil
1 teaspoon dried thyme
1 teaspoon dried basil
Salt and pepper to taste

Instructions:
- In a large pot, heat the olive oil over medium heat.
- Add the diced onion and minced garlic. Sauté for 2-3 minutes until the onion is translucent.
Stir in the shredded cabbage and cook for another 5 minutes until it begins to wilt.
- Add the diced tomatoes (with juice), vegetable broth, tomato paste, dried thyme, dried basil, salt, and pepper. Stir to combine everything.
- Bring the soup to a boil, then reduce the heat to low and simmer for 20-25 minutes until the cabbage is tender.
- Adjust the seasoning if needed. Serve hot.

SIDE DISHES

12. Crispy Fried Cabbage

Ingredients:
- 1 small cabbage, thinly sliced
- 2 tablespoons vegetable oil
- 2 cloves garlic, minced
- 1 teaspoon soy sauce
- 1/2 teaspoon sesame oil
- Salt and pepper to taste

Instructions:
- In a large skillet or wok, heat the vegetable oil over medium-high heat.
- Saute the minced garlic for 1 minute, or until aromatic.
- Add the thinly sliced cabbage to the skillet and stir-fry for 5-7 minutes until it begins to wilt and turn golden brown.
- Add the soy sauce, sesame oil, salt, and pepper to taste. Continue to cook for another 2-3 minutes until the cabbage is crispy and well-coated.
- Remove from the heat and place in a serving dish. Serve hot as a flavorful side dish.

13. Cabbage And Carrot Slaw

Ingredients:
- 1 small cabbage, thinly sliced

- 2 carrots, grated
- 1/2 cup mayonnaise
- 2 tablespoons apple cider vinegar
- 1 tablespoon honey
- 1 teaspoon Dijon mustard
- Salt and pepper to taste

Instructions:
- In a large bowl, combine the thinly sliced cabbage and grated carrots.
- In a separate bowl, combine the mayonnaise, apple cider vinegar, honey, and Dijon mustard. mustard, salt, and pepper until well-combined.
- Drizzle the dressing over the cabbage-carrot combination. Toss to coat evenly.
- Refrigerate the slaw for at least 30 minutes to allow the flavors to mingle together.
- Serve chilled as a light side dish.

14. Roasted Cabbage Wedges

Ingredients:
- 1 small head of cabbage, sliced into wedges
- 2 tablespoons olive oil
- 1 teaspoon garlic powder
- 1 teaspoon paprika
- Salt and pepper to taste

Instructions:
- Preheat the oven to 425°F (220°C).Using parchment paper, line a baking sheet.
- Arrange the cabbage wedges in a single layer on the baking sheet.
- Drizzle the olive oil over the wedges, making sure to coat them evenly.
- Combine the garlic powder, paprika, salt, and pepper in a small mixing bowl. Sprinkle the mixture over the cabbage wedges.
- Roast in the oven for 20-25 minutes until the edges are crispy and golden brown.
- Remove from the oven and let it cool slightly before serving.

15. Cabbage And Onion Gratin

Ingredients:
- 1 small cabbage, thinly sliced
- 2 onions, thinly sliced
- 1 cup shredded Gruyere cheese
- 1/2 cup breadcrumbs
- 1/4 cup grated Parmesan cheese
- 1/4 cup butter, melted
- Salt and pepper to taste

Instructions:
- Preheat the oven to 375°F (190°C). Grease a baking dish with butter.

- Layer half of the thinly sliced cabbage and onions in the baking dish. Sprinkle it with salt and pepper.
- Repeat the layers with the remaining cabbage and onions. Sprinkle it with salt and pepper again.
- In a bowl, mix together the breadcrumbs, grated Parmesan cheese, and melted butter. Sprinkle the breadcrumb mixture over the top of the cabbage and onions.
- Top with shredded Gruyere cheese.
- Bake for 30-35 minutes until the cheese is melted and the gratin is golden brown on top.
- Remove from the oven and let it cool slightly before serving.

16. Cabbage And Apple Salad

Ingredients:
- 1 small cabbage, thinly sliced
- 2 apples, thinly sliced
- 1/2 cup dried cranberries
- 1/2 cup chopped walnuts
- 1/4 cup apple cider vinegar
- 2 tablespoons honey
- 2 tablespoons olive oil
- Salt and pepper to taste

Instructions:
- In a large bowl, combine the thinly sliced cabbage, apple slices, dried cranberries, and chopped walnuts.
- In a separate bowl, whisk together the apple cider vinegar, honey, olive oil, salt, and pepper until well-mixed.
- Pour the dressing over the cabbage and apple combination. Toss to coat everything evenly.
- Let the salad sit in the refrigerator for at least 30 minutes to allow the flavors to blend.
- Serve chilled as a cool side dish.

17. Cabbage And Bacon Sauté

Ingredients:
- 1 small cabbage, thinly sliced
- 6 slices bacon, chopped
- 1 onion, thinly sliced
- 2 cloves garlic, minced
- 1 tablespoon butter
- Salt and pepper to taste

Instructions:
- In a large skillet over medium heat, sauté the chopped bacon until crispy.
- Remove the bacon from the skillet and put aside. Leave about 1 tablespoon of bacon grease in the skillet.

- Melt the butter in a separate skillet over medium heat.

- Add the thinly sliced onion and minced garlic to the skillet. Sauté for 2-3 minutes until the onion is translucent.
- Add the thinly sliced cabbage to the skillet and cook for another 5-7 minutes until it is tender-crisp.
- Add the cooked bacon and season with salt & pepper to taste.
- Cook for an additional 2-3 minutes to heat everything through.
- Remove from heat and serve hot as a savory side dish.

18. Braised Red Cabbage

Ingredients:
- 1 small red cabbage, shredded
- 1 apple, peeled, cored, and chopped
- 1 onion, thinly sliced
- 1/4 cup red wine vinegar
- 2 tablespoons brown sugar
- 2 tablespoons butter
- 1 teaspoon ground cinnamon
- Salt and pepper to taste

Instructions:
- Melt the butter in a large pot or Dutch oven over medium heat.

- Add the thinly sliced onion and chopped apple to the pot. Cook for 3-4 minutes, or until the onion softens.
- Stir in the shredded red cabbage and cook for another 5 minutes until it begins to wilt.
- Add the red wine vinegar, brown sugar, ground cinnamon, salt, and pepper to the pot. Stir to combine everything evenly.
- Cover the pot and let the cabbage simmer on low heat for 30-40 minutes until it is tender and the flavors have melded together.
- Adjust the seasoning if needed. Serve warm as a flavorful side dish.

19. Cabbage And Corn Salad

Ingredients:
- 1 small cabbage, thinly sliced
- 1 cup cooked and cooled corn kernels
- 1 red bell pepper, diced
- 1/2 cup chopped fresh cilantro
- Juice of 1 lime
- 2 tablespoons olive oil
- Salt and pepper to taste

Instructions:

- In a large bowl, combine the thinly sliced cabbage, cooked corn kernels, diced red bell pepper, and chopped cilantro.
- In a small bowl, whisk together the lime juice, olive oil, salt, and pepper until well-combined.
- Drizzle the dressing over the cabbage mixture and toss to coat evenly.
- Let the salad sit in the refrigerator for at least 30 minutes to allow the flavors to mingle.
- Serve chilled as a light side dish.

20. Cabbage And Mushroom Stir-Fry

Ingredients:

- 1 small cabbage, thinly sliced
- 8 ounces mushrooms, sliced
- 1 red onion, thinly sliced
- 2 cloves garlic, minced
- 2 tablespoons soy sauce
- 1 tablespoon hoisin sauce
- 1 tablespoon sesame oil
- Salt and pepper to taste

Instructions:

- In a large skillet or wok, heat the sesame oil over medium heat.

- Add the sliced mushrooms and cook for 5-7 minutes until they release their moisture and begin to brown.
- Stir in the minced garlic and thinly sliced red onion.
Cook for an additional 2-3 minutes, or until the onion is softened.
- Add the thinly sliced cabbage to the skillet and stir-fry for 5-7 minutes until it is tender-crisp.
- In a small bowl, whisk together the soy sauce and hoisin sauce. Pour the sauce over the cabbage mixture and toss to coat everything evenly.
- Season with salt and pepper to taste.
Cook for another 2-3 minutes to thoroughly cook everything.
- Remove from heat and serve hot as a flavorful side dish.

Enjoy these 15 delicious cabbage recipes, ranging from hearty main courses to comforting soups and delightful side dishes. They showcase the versatility of cabbage and offer a range of flavors and textures to satisfy your taste buds. Whether you're looking for a wholesome meal or a tasty accompaniment, these recipes are sure to impress.

CONCLUSION

In conclusion, these cabbage recipes offer a diverse range of options to satisfy your cravings for delicious and nutritious meals. Whether you prefer hearty main courses or comforting soups, there is something for everyone. From the flavorsome Cabbage and Beef Stir-Fry to the comforting Stuffed Cabbage Rolls and the delightful Cabbage and Chicken Stir-Fry, these main courses showcase the versatility of cabbage as a key ingredient. The Cabbage and Lentil Soup and the Cabbage and Tomato Soup provide warm and comforting options that are perfect for colder days. With these recipes, you can explore the many ways to incorporate cabbage into your cooking and enjoy its unique taste and health benefits. So, grab a head of cabbage and get ready to create mouthwatering dishes that will impress your family and friends. Whether you're a cabbage enthusiast or looking to incorporate more vegetables into your diet, these recipes are sure to delight your taste buds and leave you wanting more.

Happy cooking